T0223431

A Patient's Guide to Obstructive Sleep Apnea Syndrome

Springer Nature More Media App

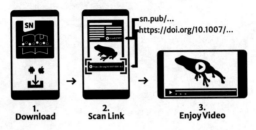

1.
Download

2.
Scan Link

3.
Enjoy Video

sn.pub/...
https://doi.org/10.1007/...

Support: customerservice@springernature.com

Arnav Shetty

Peter M Baptista Jardín

A Patient's Guide to Obstructive Sleep Apnea Syndrome

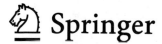 Springer

Arnav Shetty
Camperdown
Sydney, NSW, Australia

Peter M Baptista Jardín
Alzahra Hospital
Dubai, United Arab Emirates

This work contains media enhancements, which are displayed with a "play" icon. Material in the print book can be viewed on a mobile device by downloading the Springer Nature "More Media" app available in the major app stores. The media enhancements in the online version of the work can be accessed directly by authorized users.

ISBN 978-3-031-38263-5   ISBN 978-3-031-38264-2   (eBook)
https://doi.org/10.1007/978-3-031-38264-2

© The Editor(s) (if applicable) and The Author(s), under exclusive license to Springer Nature Switzerland AG 2023
This work is subject to copyright. All rights are solely and exclusively licensed by the Publisher, whether the whole or part of the material is concerned, specifically the rights of translation, reprinting, reuse of illustrations, recitation, broadcasting, reproduction on microfilms or in any other physical way, and transmission or information storage and retrieval, electronic adaptation, computer software, or by similar or dissimilar methodology now known or hereafter developed.
The use of general descriptive names, registered names, trademarks, service marks, etc. in this publication does not imply, even in the absence of a specific statement, that such names are exempt from the relevant protective laws and regulations and therefore free for general use.
The publisher, the authors, and the editors are safe to assume that the advice and information in this book are believed to be true and accurate at the date of publication. Neither the publisher nor the authors or the editors give a warranty, expressed or implied, with respect to the material contained herein or for any errors or omissions that may have been made. The publisher remains neutral with regard to jurisdictional claims in published maps and institutional affiliations.

This Springer imprint is published by the registered company Springer Nature Switzerland AG
The registered company address is: Gewerbestrasse 11, 6330 Cham, Switzerland

Paper in this product is recyclable.

I dedicate this work to my loving mother and father.

—*Arnav Shetty*

Preface

Perhaps you reached for this book out of pure curiosity, which would be slightly strange but by no means unwelcome; there's a lot in here that epitomises the spirit of medicine—a field rooted in millennia of tradition yet one that harnesses the most recent advances in science and technology. It's an inescapable priority for all intelligent life. This volume traces a salient disease affecting millions today from its earliest experimental ramblings in the ancient world to the latest surgical interventions of the present century. It will no doubt be interesting for you in this way.

If, however, you picked up this book because you think you, or a loved one, may have Obstructive Sleep Apnoea Syndrome, then allow us to be the bearers of consolation. Though it may have its romance, medicine is not easily navigable, and one can become quickly confused and frustrated by the cacophonous narratives that plague the internet and media. Your efforts might feel to have been in vain, and your anxiety deepened, and we understand. We have written this present volume precisely for you.

The fundamental issue with such a disorder is that it is highly individualised, so no two patients with the same condition would likely receive the same management strategy. The book will talk about many treatments, and at each, the question on your mind may be "well, why not just give me this one?", but the reality is that the case that concerns you is likely to be entirely unique.

Only a specialist with the right tools can plan the proper treatment. Our job is to inform you about the disorder, and we hope that you come out of it confident about your next step.

- THE AUTHORS

Arnav Shetty
Peter M Baptista Jardín

Acknowledgements

To my wife, inspiration in my life, I am so grateful for her insistence on doing this book.

To my daughters, their husbands, and grandchildren for their continuous support and admiration.

To my parents that showed me the value of hard work and effort.

To all those patients I see daily with this disease, may it serve them to have more knowledge and seek faster and adequate treatment.

—Peter M Baptista Jardin

Contents

List of Videos

An Introduction to the Field of Breathing, Circulation, and Sleep Medicine

A third of our lives is dedicated to the comfortable idleness of sleep. When we close our eyes, dream easy, and then open them to a new day, it's easy to undermine its importance. Still, the reality remains that *how* we sleep significantly affects our waking state. We all know how a bad night's sleep can throw us off kilter the next day, and a couple in a row can leave us fatigued, irritable, and unproductive. We can reverse these effects easily in the short term with some decent shuteye, but poor sleep over a long period can have some dire consequences such as a decrease in brain function, stunting of growth, decreased life expectancy, and a heightened risk of obesity, cardiovascular disease, and even cancer.

Building and maintaining good sleep habits—or sleep hygiene—is becoming a popular conversation in our modern day, where ample stress and endless distractions threaten the sanctity of our sleep. For many who find trouble getting to or staying asleep, aspects of their lifestyles such as caffeine consumption, device usage near bedtime, timing of sleep, etc., would be very worthwhile looking into.

For some, however, their troubles lie in the quality of sleep that they get. They find themselves sleeping the whole night but still waking up tired, or perhaps they are informed by their partner that they stop breathing or wake up repeatedly during sleep. This book is for these people. The other reason that we might not be getting our fair share of sleep is that we may suffer from a sleep disor-

© The Author(s), under exclusive license to Springer Nature Switzerland AG 2023
A. Shetty, P. M. Baptista Jardín, *A Patient's Guide to Obstructive Sleep Apnea Syndrome*, https://doi.org/10.1007/978-3-031-38264-2_1

der—a condition that affects, at some point, over half of the population. The prevalence of sleep disorders within the population is often underestimated because they act at a time when we are unaware and vulnerable and so take a long time to be discovered, if at all.

Although leaps and bounds are being made in diagnosing and treating sleep disorders, it remains that many of us are not having a full experience of our awake life because of a condition we may not be aware of. One in particular Obstructive Sleep Apnoea Syndrome (OSAS) will be the primary focus of this book, which aims to inform the individual who may be affected directly or indirectly by OSAS, and to guide them towards attaining the quality of life that they deserve.

1.1   Why Is Sleep So Important?

Although the importance of sleep is preached all the time in the modern day, it is still heavily neglected in the population. The quantity and quality of our sleep affect our psychological and physiological well-being, therefore directly affecting our quality of life.

What occurs during a night of sleep seems simple but is actually quite complex. It is composed of multiple different stages that come after each other in a cyclical fashion—hence why we use the term "sleep cycle". Multiple cycles occur throughout the night, and even these have a detailed structure where different stages are dominant at different times. See Fig. 1.1 for a visual representation of the evolution of sleep during the night.

It is not only important, therefore, that we sleep for a certain amount of time, but that we sleep continuously to preserve the natural structure of sleep and reap all its benefits.

There are two main stages of sleep: NREM (non-rapid eye movement) and REM (rapid eye movement) sleep. NREM sleep is further split into three stages of increasing depth, where heart rate, blood pressure, and brain activity are decreased. These stages are involved in restoring the body—the last stage is also called slow-wave or deep sleep and is the most restorative stage. After

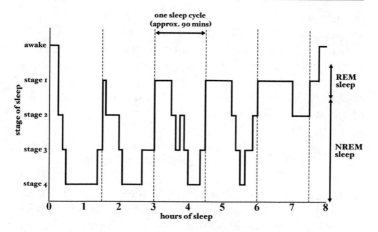

Fig. 1.1 Hypnogram demonstrating the sleep cycles

these comes REM sleep, which increases in time with each cycle, as seen in the diagram.

Although it accounts for only a fifth of overall sleeping time, it is essential for restoring the mind, especially the consolidation of memories and learning. We cycle through these stages around 4–5 times a night, each lasting around 1.5–2 h, totalling 7–9 h[1] of sleep per night for healthy adults [1].

A sufferer of OSAS may have been in bed the whole night but gain very few benefits of the sleep they've had, and that is because, as we mentioned before, a healthy sleep should be continuous and uninterrupted. OSAS is a condition that destroys the sanctity of sleep by waking the sufferer up repeatedly over the night. After every "event" of sleep apnoea, the brain needs to wake the body up to reengage the airway muscles and allow air in again, throwing the sufferer out of whatever sleep stage they may have been when it strikes. REM sleep is the stage that we are most likely to

---

[1]National Sleep Foundation's recommendations. There is the following consensus among experts: older adults should get 7–8 h of sleep per night; young adults and adults, 7–9; teenagers, 8–10; and school-aged children 9–11.

experience OSAS because the muscles in our body are relaxed, including the airway—but it can strike in any stage [2].

OSAS has a profound personal and social effect because it withholds the sufferer from regular, healthy, and restorative sleep, which is an essential part of their health. For children and teenagers, poor sleep can affect their health and development, so it is imperative that it is diagnosed early.

1.2   The Prevalence of Disturbed Sleep

According to a recent epidemiological review, between 20 and 42% of people worldwide report a consistent lack of sleep [3]. This is a startling proportion. The reasons are not always lifestyle related (e.g., caffeine intake, alcohol, sleep environment) but often are because of sleep disorders—key culprits in getting to and maintaining restorative sleep.

Sleep disordered breathing is characterised by abnormal breathing patterns during sleep and/or an overall lack of ventilation.[2] Snoring is the most prevalent sleep breathing disorder, more common among men, those who are overweight, and those of an older age. Although snoring, in general, is harmless, it could be a symptom of sleep apnoea—which is much more serious.

Within sleep disorders, sleep apnoea itself has two types: central and obstructive. Central sleep apnoea is characterised by the intermittent failure of the brain to send breathing signals to the body—a very rare condition that will not be the concern of this book. Obstructive Sleep Apnoea Syndrome (OSAS), on the other hand, is highly prevalent, taking place as the second most common sleep disorder.[3] It has been predicted that nearly a billion adults from 30 to 69 years could suffer from the condition, almost half of whom should seek treatment [4].

---

[2] Defined as the movement of air in and out of the lungs in order that the exchange of gases (oxygen and carbon dioxide) can take place.

[3] The most common being insomnia.

1.3   What Is Sleep Apnoea, and Why Should We Care About it?

Pnoea is a Greek term that means breathing, so *hypo-pnoea* and *a-pnoea* signify the reduction and stoppage of breathing, respectively. Sufferers of OSAS will completely cease breathing for 10 or more seconds at a time, and in some, more than 30 s. In severe cases, sufferers will experience these events more than 60 times an hour. During an apnoea event, the airway will collapse, creating a partial to complete seal while the lungs below are still attempting to breathe—a scary situation, no doubt.

During an apnoea, fresh oxygen is not being exchanged into the blood, so the brain, heart, and vital organs are being deprived. To stop this, the brain must wake the body to reengage the airway muscles and allow the passage of air, disturbing the sleep cycle in the process. So, when one wakes up from a night full of events of apnoea, they are not well rested and will feel sleepy throughout the day—impacting their functioning significantly.

On the whole, a sleep-deprived society does not live life to the fullest. They are not as productive and healthy as they can be and have been shown to be more dangerous on the road [5]. Sleep apnoea strikes invisibly and is tough to catch, but the good news is that it can be treated, and the advances in the field are making the diagnosis and treatment widely available.

First, we will trace the history of medicine as relevant to OSAS, focussing on the enigmas of breathing, circulation, and sleep. This is important because it highlights how central these questions about our functioning have been to human scientific thought over the millennia. Secondly, we will paint a detailed picture of OSAS itself, and lastly, discuss treatment. By the end of the book, the reader should have an informed perspective about the condition, be better equipped to deal with their own concerns, and efficiently work alongside a doctor to discuss their treatment.

References

1. Hirshkowitz M, et al. National Sleep Foundation's sleep time duration recommendations: methodology and results summary. Sleep Health. 2015;1:40–3. https://doi.org/10.1016/j.sleh.2014.12.010.
2. Strollo PJ Jr, Rogers RM. Obstructive sleep apnea. N Engl J Med. 1996;334:99–104. https://doi.org/10.1056/NEJM199601113340207.
3. Ohayon MM. Epidemiological overview of sleep disorders in the general population. Sleep Med Res. 2011;2:1–9. https://doi.org/10.17241/smr.2011.2.1.1.
4. Benjafield AV, et al. Estimation of the global prevalence and burden of obstructive sleep apnoea: a literature-based analysis. Lancet Respir Med. 2019;7:687–98. https://doi.org/10.1016/S2213-2600(19)30198-5.
5. Howard ME, et al. Sleepiness, sleep-disordered breathing, and accident risk factors in commercial vehicle drivers. Am J Respir Crit Care Med. 2004;170:1014–21. https://doi.org/10.1164/rccm.200312-1782OC.

A Brief History of Breathing and Sleep Medicine

2.1   Where It All Began: The Ancient World and the Middle Ages

As beautifully put by Dr. Alfred P. Fishman, Emeritus Professor of Medicine at the University of Pennsylvania:

> *The history of the pulmonary circulation provides a measure of Man's thinking about himself and his place in the Universe.*

For many thinkers throughout history, the specific roles of the lungs and the heart were impossible to explain and so the exact nature of how they worked together remained a mystery until approximately the seventeenth century CE. Almost every ancient society and religion has pondered on the phenomenon of breathing and circulation so the history of this area of human exploration is incredibly diverse. The book of Genesis in the Holy Bible, for example, incorporates this same theme into the creation of man:

> *Then the LORD God formed a man from the dust of the ground and breathed into his nostrils the breath of life, and the man became a living being.*[1]

---

[1] From Genesis 2:7 NIV.

© The Author(s), under exclusive license to Springer Nature Switzerland AG 2023
A. Shetty, P. M. Baptista Jardín, *A Patient's Guide to Obstructive Sleep Apnea Syndrome*, https://doi.org/10.1007/978-3-031-38264-2_2

It was not only in the Bible that breathing was seen in a divine light, as we will see shortly. It was the strange nature of the "beating" heart or the invisibility of the air that we breathed that might have inspired such radical notions, or perhaps it was just the complexity of a deceptively simple process that left these thinkers utterly clueless.

We know now that the heart is a double pump: deoxygenated[2] blood from the body comes into the right side of the heart, where it is pumped into the lungs to be reoxygenated and for carbon dioxide to be removed (see Fig. 2.1). This fresh blood leaves the lungs and arrives at the left side of the heart, where it is pumped into the body to deliver nutrients and oxygen to all our tissues. When these have been used up and the oxygen is replaced by carbon dioxide (a waste product), it returns into the right side of the heart, and the cycle continues—clearly not the simplest concept.

The earliest sign of understanding comes from the ancient Egyptians, who evidently had a keen interest in the practice and scholarship of medicine throughout their existence. We can gather from scant evidence in the form of papyri from 3500 to 1500 BCE that they made a connection between the heartbeat and the pulse in the wrist, and notably believed that there was a system of vessels throughout the body that distributed important elements and nutrients, including air.[3] This is significant, as the connection between the heart, circulation, and air is a difficult one, and a very important step. They did not explore much further by means of dissection of the human body, so their knowledge remained there [1, 2].

The Greeks, a couple centuries later, began to philosophise in all fields of knowledge, including medicine and anatomy. The Milesian philosopher Anaximenes[4] concluded that *aer* (air), or

---

[2]Depleted of oxygen, as the body used the oxygen from the blood to make energy.

[3]The Edwin Smith (1750 BCE) and Ebers (1500 BCE) papyri are most significant.

[4]Born in Miletus (present-day Turkey) in the sixth century BCE. One of the first western philosophers.

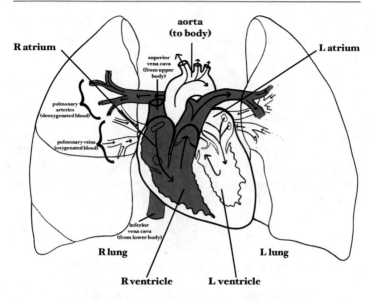

Fig. 2.1 Pulmonary circulation
A rather interesting design. Regions in grey represent "deoxygenated" blood returning to the heart from the body. Note how it enters the heart via the inferior vena cava (blood from lower limbs and abdomen) and the superior vena cava (blood from the head, neck, and upper limbs). This blood passes through the right side of the heart and is pumped through the lungs where it becomes "oxygenated" again. Now, it collects from the lungs in the left side of the heart, and is pumped to the whole body via the aorta, which has many branches heading in many directions. The blood then serves its purpose and returns again to the right side of the heart

pneuma—a wide term encompassing breathed air, breath of life, and divine spirit—was not only the raw ingredient of all things, but also the stuff that circulated in our arteries and veins. It was this substance, according to the Greeks, that was breathed in and out of our bodies, and that distributed *vital heat*, an innate quantity that gives rise to life.

Ancient theories on respiration strongly upheld the notion that either the brain or the heart was the centre of the soul and was where air went when we breathed. Another important Greek from the fourth century BCE known as Hippocrates,[5] considered the father of medicine, even studied the periodicity of breathing but made no connection with the lungs. Over the next few centuries, cardiocentrist[6] thinking began to dominate, and various philosophers uncovered some pieces of the puzzle that would aid later thinkers,[7] such as the discovery of cardiac valves, the two sides of the heart, and the movement of substance between the heart and lungs [3].

Half a millennium later, another legendary Greek physician, Galen,[8] who wrote prolifically and served many early Roman emperors, described in detail the anatomy and physiology of the thorax but was still unable to explain the nature of pulmonary circulation.

Unfortunately, Galen was the last great mind to concern themself with this topic for another millennium and a half. A lack of further understanding of anatomy and physics hampered the advancement of this field, and the adoption of the ancient findings into Christian doctrine gave them a certain irrefutability that remained unchallenged for a long time [4].

2.2   The Renaissance of Breathing Medicine: Fifteenth to Eighteenth Centuries

The western world only revisited this problem during the Renaissance. In his detailed depiction of the human heart, Leonardo da Vinci (1452–1519) correctly noted all the structures we see today, including valves and coronary arteries. Though there was no physical evidence of blood passing between the

---

[5] Born on the island of Cos, Greece, in the fourth century BCE. Considered the "father of modern medicine", as his life's work laid many pillars of the field of medicine into the modern day, such as the importance of scientific reasoning and ethics in the practice in medicine.

[6] That is, believing that the heart was the seat of the soul, mind, and body.

[7] Such as Plato and his student Aristotle, in the late fourth century BCE, and Herophilus and his student Erasistratus in the third century BCE.

[8] Born in Pergamon (present-day Turkey) in the second century BCE.

chambers as per the Galenic theory, he was nevertheless convinced of it and so attributed it to invisible pores [4].

It was only in the sixteenth century that the first accurate representation of pulmonary circulation was found. It is debated as to exactly who and when, but most attribute the discovery to the renowned Spanish polymath Michael Serveto (c.1511–1553), who reported it in his magnum opus, the *Christianismi Restitutio*. The western world is specified, as the Arab world actually received an accurate theory of pulmonary circulation and capillary anatomy almost three centuries earlier from the physician and prolific scholar Ibn Al-Nafis, in his *Commentary on Anatomy in Avicenna's Canon* [5]. Though his legacy and work strongly influenced later Islamic scholarship, it did not surface in the western world until the early twentieth century. Michel Serveto's independent discovery that blood actually passes via the lungs rather than just between the chambers of the heart and also that the blood in the pulmonary vein is mixed with air were the fundamental notions that motivated a renaissance in the science of breathing [5].

Later that century, physicians Andreas Vesalius (1514–1564) and Realdo Colombo (1516–1559), prominent anatomists from the Paduan School of Medicine (the centre of western medical research at the time) confirmed Serveto's findings as they were unable to find the perforations between the chambers of the heart. A century later, the work of William Harvey[9] and Marcello Malpighi[10] built on this, helping codify a near-modern description of blood circulation [4].

It's quite understandable why the complicated phenomenon of respiration and circulation has confounded thinkers for generations. Though circulation was described quite well, the role of breathing and oxygen took much longer. Understanding why we breathe, however, was the next great challenge in this field.

---

[9]Born in Kent, England, 1579 d. London, England 1657. Prominent physician and anatomist who very precisely described the route of blood around the body.

[10]Born in Crevalcore, Papal States, 1628, died in Rome, Papal States, 1694. Prominent physician and scientist. Considered the founder of histology, a study of body tissues on a microscopic level.

In the seventeenth century, four Oxford researchers, Robert Boyle, Robert Hooke, John Locke, and John Mayow, showed that air must be necessary for life, air is mixed with blood in the lungs, and that there is a specific part of air that is vital. This specific part was discovered in the eighteenth century by Carl Wilhelm Scheele[11] and Joseph Priestley[12] independently, and later renamed from *vital air* to *oxygen* by the Frenchman Antoine-Laurent Lavoisier[13] in 1777 [3].

2.3   Late Nineteenth to the Late Twentieth Century

OSAS is the intersection between the physical mechanisms of breathing and the mysterious subtleties of the state of sleep. As we have discussed, the former was mainly studied by anatomical exploration, but characterising sleep was much more subtle and required new techniques. Prior to the twentieth century, dreams were more of interest than sleep itself, but this is understandable as the study of sleep was only accessible with the advent of technology such as electricity.

In 1875, Englishman Richard Caton[14] reported to the *British Medical Journal* that there is indeed electrical activity in the

---

[11] Born in Stralsund, Swedish Pomerania, 1786, Scheele was a German-Swedish chemist who, along with oxygen, identified many other elements and compounds such as tungsten, chlorine, lactic acid, and glycerol.

[12] Born in Yorkshire, England, 1733, Priestley was an English polymath, with achievements in the fields of political theory, grammar, theology, and, as is relevant presently, chemistry. He is credited with the discovery of the carbon cycle, as well as the discovery of multiple gases in addition to oxygen such as ammonia and carbon monoxide.

[13] Born in Paris, 1743, Lavoisier was a prolific chemist, changing the direction of the field. He is also credited with the naming of hydrogen and the prediction of silicon.

[14] Born in Bradford, England, 1842, Caton was a physician whose work, along with the later work of the German psychiatrist Hans Berger (born in the German Empire, 1873), led to the description of brain waves (rhythmic electrical oscillations in the brain), most prominently Alpha waves, which led to the invention of the electroencephalogram.

brains of animals during sleep, which he measured using a volt-meter. Furthering his work, Hans Berger first explored the electrical activity of a human brain in 1924 and produced the first EEG (electroencephalogram[15]) [6]. This would later be used in a polysomnography, the state-of-the-art diagnostic test for patients with potential OSAS. Another critical part of this test is eye movement, which is used to help determine which stage of sleep the patient is in at any given time. We experience both REM (rapid eye movement) and NREM (non-rapid eye movement) sleep during the night. There is a remarkable difference in the activity of our body, and consequence due to their loss when we are awake. This phenomenon, along with many other groundbreaking observations within the science of sleep, was presented by Nathaniel Kleitmann[16] and his team at Chicago University. Their contributions to the science of sleep have been vital to the state of modern sleep science.

Simultaneously, understanding the relationship between breathing and gas concentration in the blood started to develop during the early twentieth century when Scottish physiologist John Scott Haldane[17] described the gas exchange process in red blood cells as they passed through the lung. He also described the need to breath when we detect that the concentration of carbon dioxide gets too high in the blood [7].

---

[15]A graphical representation of the brain's electrical activity. It is generated by attaching multiple electrodes along the scalp of the patient and monitoring the electrical signals arising from them.

[16]Born in Kishinev, Russian Empire, 1899, Nathaniel Kleitmann was an American physiologist fascinated by the body and brain's activity during sleep. His work propelled sleep physiology into a major field of scientific research.

[17]Born in Edinburgh, Scotland, 1860, Hadlane was a Scottish physician who, along with describing the mentioned gas exchange process in red blood cells (specifically the reduced affinity for carbon dioxide binding in haemoglobin with the increase of oxygen concentration, known as the Hadlane effect), is credited with the invention of the respirator, which was used by soldiers in World War 1.

As knowledge in these fields grew, a relationship between sleep and breathing slowly became evident. In the mid-twentieth century, an association between poor ventilation and obesity was described [8], and it was especially noticed around the mid-1960s that the recurrent collapse of the upper airway during sleep disrupted its therapeutic function, leading to daytime sleepiness. This was the first description of the topic of this book: Obstructive Sleep Apnoea Syndrome [9]. The concurrent advances in the understanding of sleep and its importance skyrocketed this area into a global effort: William Dement, a student of Nathaniel Kleitmann, established the first sleep clinic in Stanford University, USA, and research into respiratory sleep disorders was soon commenced, with 381 papers being published between 1975 and 80 on this topic.

2.4   Late Twentieth Century to the Modern Day

Until 1981, the primary treatments for OSAS were weight loss or tracheostomy (a hole is made in the windpipe to breathe from, bypassing the blockage higher up), which were both quite complex solutions.[18] In this year at Sydney University, Colin E. Sullivan published a paper that introduced an effective treatment for certain patients with a history of snoring and excessive daytime sleepiness: Continuous Positive Airway Pressure (CPAP). This will be elaborated on in a further section. Still, the invention was very significant in the field, as the technology alleviates many of the symptoms of the condition and is still in common use today [10].

The introduction of the CPAP treatment strategy in sufferers of OSAS was not without difficulty, however. Many did not tolerate

---

[18]Weight loss requires lifestyle changes that are often difficult to implement, especially for those feel unenergetic and unmotivated during the day because of their poor sleep. A tracheostomy affects the patient's quality of life by complicating daily activities such as speaking and eating. This procedure is described in Chap. 5.

the treatment, so various surgical procedures were developed to treat the condition directly or make CPAP more tolerable.

During the mid-1980s, a procedure called Uvulopalatopharyngoplasty became very popular in treating OSAS. This surgery included the modification of the back of the throat and the uvula to open it up (discussed in detail in Chap. 5). Although this procedure stopped many patients from snoring, it only improved the OSAS of a small group of patients[19] and caused some unwanted side effects in those who had it, such as unnatural sensations and food entering the nose when swallowing.

Over the next decade, the Stanford group mentioned above developed various maxillofacial procedures (surgically adjusting the structure of the bones around the mouth) for those who did not tolerate the popular surgical interventions. Still, these were generally restricted to patients that have deformities of the facial skeleton, issues with the alignment of their teeth, or nasal problems.

More conservative procedures began to be developed during the mid-2000s to open up the airway without annoying post-surgical side effects. For those whose tongues fell back into the throat during sleep causing OSAS, the partial reduction of the size of the tongue was an effective procedure and often accompanied uvulopalatopharyngoplasty. In the modern day, a recently developed procedure called Hypoglossal Nerve Stimulation bypasses the need for reducing the tongue by stimulating the nerve that controls the tongue whenever the sleeping patient breathes in, causing it to move forward and out of the airway. This treatment was FDA approved in 2014 and has had excellent results. It is elaborated on in Chap. 5 of this book.

Recently, non-invasive treatments and devices are becoming popular such as Mandibular Advancement Devices, which are put in the mouth during sleep and hold the airway open physically. They are only applicable (and to a varying degree of success) for snorers and those with mild to medium OSAS. These recent advancements will also be dealt with in detail in Chap. 4 of this book.

---

[19]Those with large tonsils, a large mouth opening, and no tongue collapse. Such features are very common among OSAS sufferers.

2.5 To Conclude..

For the last two and a half millennia, humans have been intrigued by the nature of breathing and circulation—its exploration has progressed closely alongside the development of human thought and intellectual learning. Sleep, equally, has been as much the subject of scientific bafflement as it has a muse for poets. Sleep breathing, being a union of these important parts of our history, must therefore have our full appreciation, and any disorder that may affect it, our full scrutiny.

As we arrive at the modern day, however, we find ourselves in a most fortunate position. Not only do we have a trove of scientific and clinical knowledge to base our treatments on, but we live in an age where rapidly developing technology is making interventions safer, more accessible, more effective, and most importantly better tailored to our individual needs. Patients with OSAS should not worry; instead, they should aim to educate themselves about the condition and take the proper steps to treatment and a better quality of life.

References

1. Bestetti RB, Restini CB, Couto LB. Development of anatomophysiologic knowledge regarding the cardiovascular system: from Egyptians to Harvey. Arq Bras Cardiol. 2014;103:538–45. https://doi.org/10.5935/abc.20140148.
2. Willerson JT, T. R. Egyptian contributions to cardiovascular medicine. Tex Heart Inst J. 1996;23:191–200.
3. Fitting JW. From breathing to respiration. Respiration. 2015;89:82–7. https://doi.org/10.1159/000369474.
4. ElMaghawry M, Zanatta A, Zampieri F. The discovery of pulmonary circulation: from Imhotep to William Harvey. Glob Cardiol Sci Pract. 2014;2014:103–16. https://doi.org/10.5339/gcsp.2014.31.
5. West JB. Ibn al-Nafis, the pulmonary circulation, and the Islamic Golden age. J Appl Physiol. 2008;1985(105):1877–80. https://doi.org/10.1152/japplphysiol.91171.2008.
6. Dement WC. The study of human sleep: a historical perspective. Thorax. 1998;53(Suppl 3):S2–7.

7. Sekhar K, Rao SC. John Scott Haldane: the father of oxygen therapy. Indian J Anaesth. 2014;58:350–2. https://doi.org/10.4103/0019-5049.135087.
8. Bickelmann AG, Burwell CS, Robin ED, Whaley RD. Extreme obesity associated with alveolar hypoventilation; a Pickwickian syndrome. Am J Med. 1956;21:811–8. https://doi.org/10.1016/0002-9343(56)90094-8.
9. Gastaut H, Tassinari CA, Duron B. Polygraphic study of the episodic diurnal and nocturnal (hypnic and respiratory) manifestations of the Pickwick syndrome. Brain Res. 1966;1:167–86. https://doi.org/10.1016/0006-8993(66)90117-x.
10. Sullivan CE, Issa FG, Berthon-Jones M, Eves L. Reversal of obstructive sleep apnoea by continuous positive airway pressure applied through the nares. Lancet. 1981;1:862–5. https://doi.org/10.1016/s0140-6736(81)92140-1.

A Description of Obstructive Sleep Apnoea Syndrome: Its Nature and Diagnosis

3

The most famous literary case of sleep disordered breathing is the fat boy Joe from Dickens' first novel *The Pickwick Papers,*

> *'Sleep!' said the old gentleman, 'he's always asleep. Goes on errands fast asleep, and snores as he waits at table.'*
> *'How very odd!' said Mr. Pickwick.*
> *'Ah! odd indeed,' returned the old gentleman; 'I'm proud of that boy— wouldn't part with him on any account—he's a natural curiosity!'*

Dickens often based characters on real-life people he met, and the condition this poor boy had was what we now know as Obesity Hypoventilation Syndrome, or Pickwickian Syndrome, which is closely related to sleep apnoea [1]. The boy, because of the structure of his neck, couldn't breathe effectively enough during sleep, and therefore was sleepy throughout the day. It was certainly easy to pass off as a curiosity, and many sufferers who shared Joe's trait wouldn't receive clinical help until more than a 100 years after they might have sympathised with him in reading the book.

Thankfully, we have a much better way of describing and diagnosing this disorder, which will be explored in this chapter.

Supplementary Information The online version contains supplementary material available at https://doi.org/10.1007/978-3-031-38264-2_3. The videos can be accessed individually by clicking the DOI link in the accompanying figure caption or by scanning this link with the SN More Media App.

© The Author(s), under exclusive license to Springer Nature Switzerland AG 2023
A. Shetty, P. M. Baptista Jardín, *A Patient's Guide to Obstructive Sleep Apnea Syndrome*, https://doi.org/10.1007/978-3-031-38264-2_3

3.1   Types of Sleep Apnoea

Sleep apnoea can be obstructive, central, or mixed (both). Intermittent periods of no breathing lasting 10 s or more are present in both, but in obstructive apnoea the body tries to breathe but fails, as the collapse of the tissues of the upper airway (the base of the tongue, soft palate, and the walls of the throat) obstructs airflow into the lungs (see Figs. 3.1 and 3.2). In central apnoea, however, there is no respiratory effort because the brain fails to send a message for the person to breathe. Sufferers can present with either or both, which is called complex or mixed sleep apnoea.

An "event" is defined as either an *apnoea*[1] (caused by complete obstruction of the airway for more than 10 s) or a *hypopnoea*[2] (caused by partial obstruction of the airway for more than 10 s). The severity of a person's sleep apnoea can be roughly determined by the number of apnoea or hypopnoea events that occur per hour and is called the apnoea-hypopnoea index, or AHI.

The AHI system played an essential role during the development of OSAS research, as it helped differentiate the disorder from other similar disorders and compare treatments (an effective treatment decreases a patient's AHI). It should however be kept in mind that the AHI system is rather arbitrary; patients with low AHIs may have severe symptoms, while those with severe OSAS may be asymptomatic. Though still widely used, its appropriateness as a modern and rigorous clinical tool is declining [2].

An AHI of less than 5 is considered normal in adults, and 30 and above is severe. The necessity and type of treatment can be decided according to the following table.

AHI	Severity
Less than 5	Normal
5–14	Mild
15–29	Moderate
30 or greater	Severe

---

[1] Greek for: "no breathing".
[2] Greek for: "reduced breathing".

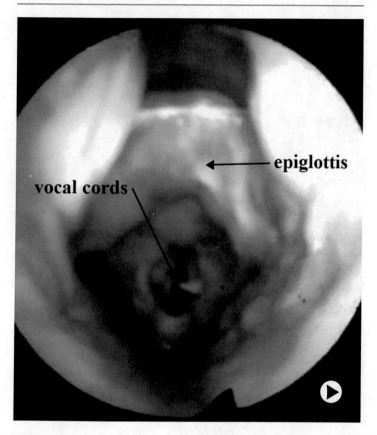

Fig. 3.1 DISE 1 (▶ https://doi.org/10.1007/000-b7r)

This value, along with other information such as body position, oxygen concentration in the blood, and eye movement, is determined during a sleep test, or polysomnography.

It's important to remember that the AHI does not necessarily define how the patient is affected by the disease. In some cases, a patient with a high AHI may have no important symptoms of OSAS. On the other hand, a patient with a low AHI may exhibit many symptoms.

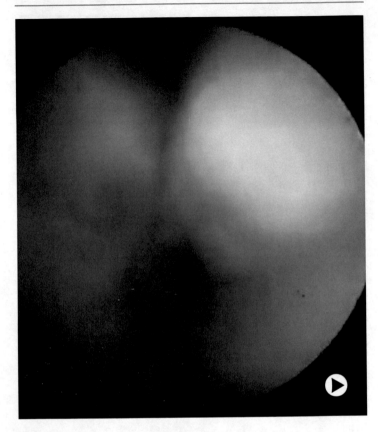

Fig. 3.2   DISE 2 (▶ https://doi.org/10.1007/000-b7q)
Images of an apnoea event taken during a DISE (drug-induced sleep endoscopy); a link to the full video is included in Chap. 6 (Video 6.1). The patient is sedated in order to simulate sleep, and a scope is inserted through the nose to visualise the upper airway. In Fig. 3.1, the airway is open and unobstructed, so air can pass through freely. You can see the vocal cords at the bottom and the epiglottis too. In Fig. 3.2, the airway has collapsed during an apnoea event. This, as can be seen, completely obstructs the flow of air

3.2   The Anatomy of Obstructive Sleep Apnoea[3]

An apnoea is caused by the collapse of the upper airway, which restricts the passage of air into the lungs. Humans are the only natural[4] species in the animal kingdom to experience sleep apnoea, and understanding our anatomy helps determine why.

After passing through the nose and mouth, inhaled air enters the throat—or pharynx—which is a complex structure due to its many responsibilities. Air then gushes through the windpipe—or trachea—to the lung via the bronchial tree, finally reaching the alveoli, where gas exchange between air and the blood circulation occurs (see Fig. 3.3).

Many of the issues with OSAS occur in the pharynx, so we will discuss them to some detail.

The pharynx is a complex and multifunctional organ with many moving parts. Firstly, it must reliably allow air to pass through it—a requirement ever since vertebrates started to live out of water. Secondly, it must conduct food and water and ensure that they do not enter where the air is supposed to go (the trachea). Lastly, it must house the complex and fascinating structures that create sound.

During man's anatomic evolution, after we started to stand upright, our pharynx descended from a high position to work with the jaw in creating the spaces required for the amplification and modification of sound. The anatomical changes made to produce sound also caused problems for us. Some of these are elaborated below:

- A reduction of the jaw and increased freedom of movement meant more complex sounds to be made. Still, it also can fall backward and restrict breathing and swallowing during sleep.

---

[3]This section is largely for those who are particularly interested. It can be skipped without majorly compromising one's understanding of OSAS.

[4]Certain species of miniature pig [3] and bulldog [4] also experience the condition.

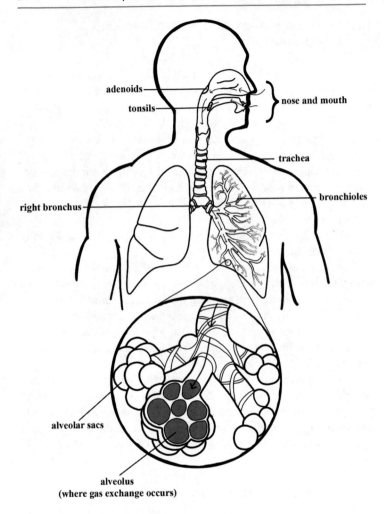

Fig. 3.3 Path of air through the body
Outside air enters the body through the nose and mouth. It then passes the structures in the upper airway such as the base of the tongue, the tonsils, and the larynx (or voice box). It then passes down a 10 cm tube called the trachea which is kept sturdy by rings of cartilage. Once the trachea enters the chest, it bifurcates into the "bronchi", which then continue to fork and divide through the lungs, eventually reaching microscopic sacs called alveoli, which are richly surrounded by blood in small vessels called capillaries. This is where oxygen is absorbed into the blood and carbon dioxide is expelled, to then be breathed out

- A right-angled connection of the mouth/nose and the throat helps us stand upright but makes the oral cavity smaller and causes our teeth to crowd (why we often don't have space for our wisdom teeth).
- A large tongue that occupies more than just the oral cavity (as in other animals), but which can collapse backward and block the airway.
- The elimination of overlap between the soft palate and epiglottis.
- A floating hyoid bone that supports the structures in the lower pharynx.

OSAS can almost be considered as the price we must pay for the ability to speak—something that has no doubt been central in our development as a species.

3.3   Risk Factors for Obstructive Sleep Apnoea

Though OSAS can present in anyone, there are certain predisposing factors; for example: if you are male, have a high body-mass index, and are of advanced age, you are at the highest risk.

Those also at heightened risk are those with a family history of the condition [5], non-Caucasians, those with an abnormal craniofacial anatomy,[5] and those who smoke/drink alcohol [6]. Each of these risk factors will be elaborated upon.

3.3.1   Gender

Men are around 3 times more likely to have sleep disordered breathing than women. Still, OSAS has a different prevalence depending on the source of data: a ratio of 5–8:1 is observed in clinics, whereas 2–3:1 is seen when surveying the population.

---

[5]The shape of the face and jaw. Some people have a naturally more congested airway and so are at a higher risk of OSAS. Facial shape is genetic, so these characteristics can travel to the next generation.

Understanding the reason for the disparity is essential, as it may help reduce the underdiagnosis of females with OSAS. Females are less likely to present with the loud and obvious symptoms of sleep apnoea, usually reporting less dramatic symptoms such as fatigue and tiredness. Furthermore, males are less likely to report irregularities in their partner's sleep activity, so OSAS in women tends to remain undiagnosed for longer. Women reaching menopause are also more prone to experience OSAS because of the hormonal imbalance and weight gain typical during this period [5].

3.3.2   Age

The prevalence of OSAS increases significantly with age until around 65, where it plateaus. As aforementioned, some advanced age groups have shown that up to 90% of men and 78% of women have mild to severe sleep apnoea [6].

3.3.3   Excessive Weight

Excessive weight and obesity are strongly linked to the risk of OSAS. The distribution of fat around the body causes a twofold restriction on the airway. Firstly, fat takes up space, which can impinge on the area that air needs to go. In the upper airway, fat around the throat can directly crowd the airway, and lower abdominal fat can compress the lungs and pressure the airway from below. Secondly, excess fat cells in the neck are thought to affect the neural signals that control respiration, further hindering sleep breathing. Decreasing weight[6] has been strongly linked to a decrease in the severity of OSAS [7].

---

[6]The prevalence of sleep apnoea for those with a BMI greater than 40 kg/m^2 has been found to be almost 90%, and a 10% change in body weight has been linked with nearly 30% change in AHI.

3.3.4   Smoking and Alcohol

Both factors put the healthy person at greater risk of developing sleep apnoea and worsen existing sleep apnoea. Those with a high alcohol intake are 25% more likely to develop OSAS. The mechanism is not clearly known but thought to be linked to its effect on the tongue's muscle tone (making it more prone to collapsing during sleep) and to dietary factors. Similarly, smoking potentially inflames the upper airway, alters muscular function, and interferes with the structure of sleep [8, 9]. There is not yet enough evidence to comment definitively on the effect of e-cigarettes and other tobacco substitutes on sleep apnoea.

Though lifestyle and genetic factors can strongly predispose certain people to the disease, it is reiterated that OSAS can present in anyone, even those who don't have the listed risk factors.

3.4   The Diagnosis of Obstructive Sleep Apnoea

Snoring is the first symptom commonly noticed, usually by partners, that may indicate sleep apnoea. Though all cases of snoring do not present with obstructive sleep apnoea, almost all patients that present with apnoea snore (~95%) [10]. Snoring is a nocturnal symptom, and below is a list of more nocturnal and daytime symptoms of the condition.

Nocturnal symptoms	Description
Audible sleep disturbances	Usually noticed by partners, such as choking, stoppage of breathing, heavy snoring, gasping, etc.
Frequent arousals	Often noticed in either the sufferers themselves or their partners. Remember that the body needs to wake up to stop the apnoea
Sexual dysfunction and impotence	Sleep apnoea has been linked with erectile dysfunction in men [10]

Daytime symptom	Description
Dry mouth and morning headaches	Short duration morning headaches are reported in up to 50% of OSAS sufferers [11]
Excessive daytime fatigue and sleepiness	Constant sleepiness during the day and dissatisfaction with sleep. The feeling of fatigue is characterised by the feeling of a lack of energy to engage in activities
Decreased cognitive ability	Poorer attention and long-term memory function [12]
Weight gain, personality changes, depression	Long-term sleep deficit as a result of OSAS has had these effects [13]

Suppose one notices these changes and comes into a clinic. In that case, preliminary tests will be carried out to rule out other possibilities. A verbal discussion of the symptoms will generally be complemented with a subjective sleep analysis via a questionnaire such as the STOP-BANG, STOP, Berlin Questionnaire (BQ), or the Epworth Sleepiness Scale (ESS). According to multiple systematic reviews, the STOP-BANG and STOP questionnaires are the most appropriate screening tools to determine those likely to have OSAS. The Berlin Questionnaire was more effective for those with a more severe condition and found to be less consistent than other screening tools, and the ESS has been shown to be unable to distinguish snorers from those with OSAS [6, 14–17].

On the next page (Fig. 3.4) we have an example of the STOP-BANG and an ESS questionnaire adapted from the original authors Chung et al. (2008) and Johns (1991) [15, 18]. Note that the STOP Questionnaire is essentially the same, but with open fields for the following categories, which replace the BANG section:

1. Height (cm).
2. Weight (kg).
3. Age.
4. Male/Female.

5. BMI (kg).
6. Collar size of shirt (S, M, L, XL, or cm).
7. Neck circumference (cm).

These questionnaires, especially the STOP and STOP-BANG, are excellent screening tools to stratify a patient's needs with potential OSAS.

Next, a physical examination will be done. Since OSAS is an upper airway disease, a thorough examination by an otolaryngologist or sleep physician is preferred. A multidisciplinary team should be employed for a diagnosis, however, as input from GPs and specialists in the lungs, heart, internal medicine, etc. are valuable for an accurate diagnosis and a personalised treatment plan.

The physical examination can be split into five parts, as follows:

General Examination
A high body-mass index is common among those diagnosed. Obese (BMI ≥ 30) and overweight (BMI 25–30) patients are at most significant risk, but OSAS can present in those of normal weight as well [19].

Neck circumference correlates well to risk of OSAS: for males, >44 cm and >41 cm for females are the risk thresholds [19].

Facial Skeleton
Abnormalities in the facial structure may signify a greater OSAS risk. The face profile can be determined by examining the relative position of the upper and lower jaws. Since they move a lot, this region's healthy bone and soft tissue structure are vital for unobstructed airflow.

Nose
The nose is a complicated structure that is responsible for up to 50% of the upper airway resistance. After observing the general shape of the nose and the size of the nostrils, the clinician will open the nostril and visually examine the front part of the

a

Please answer the following with a yes/no to determine whether you may be at risk of having Obstructive Sleep Apnoea Syndrome.

Snoring: Do you snore loudly (louder than talking or loud enough to be heard through closed doors)?

Tired: Do you often feel tired, fatigued, or sleepy during the daytime?

Observed: Has anyone observed you stop breathing during sleep?

Pressure: Do you have, or are you being treated for, high blood pressure?

Body-Mass index: Is your BMI greater than 35kg/m²?

Age: Are you above 50 years old?

Neck Circumference:

Gender:

High risk of OSAS: 3+ "yes" responses, otherwise low risk.

Fig. 3.4 An example of the STOP-BANG (**a**) and ESS (**b**) questionnaire

b

How likely are you to doze off or fall asleep in the following situations, in contrast to just feeling tired? This refers to your usual way of life in recent times. Even if you have not done some of these things recently, try to consider how they would have affected you.

Use the following scale to select the most appropriate number for each scenario:

0 = would *never* doze off
1 = *slight* chance of dozing off
2 = *moderate* chance of dozing off
3 = *high* chance of dozing off

Situation	**Chance of dozing**
Sitting and reading	
Watching TV	_____
Sitting, inactive in a public place (e.g. a theatre or a meeting)	_____
As a passenger in a car for an hour without a break	_____
Lying down to rest in the afternoon when circumstances permit	_____
Sitting and talking to someone	_____
Sitting quietly after a lunch without alcohol	_____
In a car, stopped for a few minutes in the traffic	_____

A score of greater than 10 may indicate excessive daytime sleepiness, and it is suggested to see a specialist.

Fig. 3.4 (continued)

nose. To examine further inside, the clinician will need the help of an endoscope to examine the internal structure of the naso and oropharynx (back of the nose and the throat). Common issues are a deviated septum, enlarged turbinates, or nasal polyps as pictured, which physically obstruct the passage of air (see Fig. 3.5).

Tongue and Mouth

By looking in the mouth, the clinician can note the proximity of the tongue to the soft palate and give it a scoring such as the Mallampati score. This value is very relevant as each point increase more than doubles the risk of OSAS and increases the AHI by more than 5 [20]. A high-arched palate and the thickness of the hard palate are also risk factors, as they contribute to narrowness and congestion of the nose.

Throat (Oropharynx)

Next along the path of air flow is the throat, which can be examined by looking inside the mouth and with an endoscope through the nose. The entrance of the mouth to the throat is obstructed by the back of the tongue and the tonsils. Based on the size of these structures and their relation to their surroundings, the contribution of this region to the overall obstruction can be determined by a Friedman score (Fig. 3.6). By considering this, the clinician can better predict the effectiveness of surgery or issues that may arise in using CPAP.

Enlarged tonsils can obstruct the airway but are not always obvious when looking in the throat of a sitting patient. In some cases, the tonsils only block the airway when the patient is lying down, which should be assessed.

It is also important to check the back of the throat as it extends below the level of the tongue. The base of the tongue and epiglottis (a flap that blocks off the airway when we swallow) should be checked for any abnormalities via endoscopy.

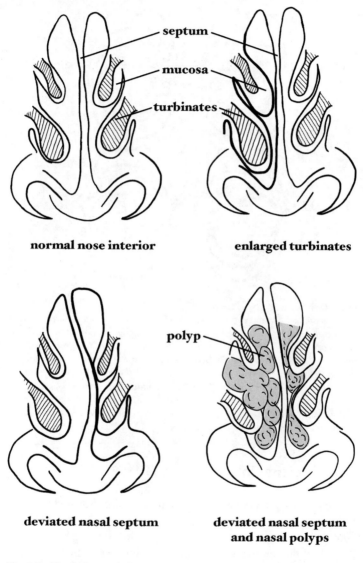

Fig. 3.5 Nasal obstructions
This particular view is front-on, but if the skin were removed. You can still see the tip of the nose and the nostrils. Note the different abnormalities that can obstruct the passage of air. You can be born with a deviated septum, but the enlarged turbinates and mucosa often are caused by allergies or infections

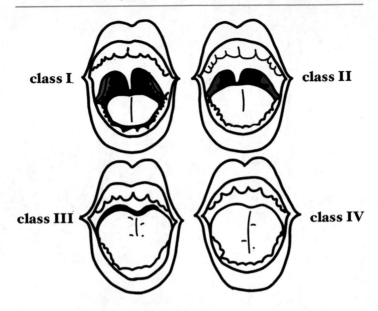

Fig. 3.6 Friedman tongue score
The Friedman tongue score is conducted by asking the patient to relax their tongue and keep it inside their mouth. It is a modified version of the Mallampati score, which is done with the tongue extended outside the mouth. These tests aim to quicky identify the distance between the palate and the tongue and therefore how difficult it is for air to travel through the mouth into the back of the throat. Notice that for a class I individual, there is a big, open space, but for a class IV, the tongue and palate are so close together than air that very little air can get through. This type of patient likely has obstructive sleep apnoea syndrome

3.5   Further Investigations: DISE

There are complementary exams that may be performed to better understand anatomical factors that may obstruct the area and compromise the airway. A DISE (Drug-Induced Sleep Endoscopy) is a study that allows an examination while the patient is asleep using a drug or combination of drugs.

The DISE was first performed in the UK in 1991 as a faster and cheaper alternative to performing endoscopy during the night under natural sleep. The patient is put to sleep for a short, controlled period with a drug, or combination of drugs (such as propofol, midazolam, or dexmedetomidine) and their airway is observed. The method is somewhat controversial as the sleep is technically not natural, but computers are used to administer a precisely controlled dose of sedative as to mimic non-REM sleep as close as possible. Close similarities in the respiratory activity of natural sleep have been noted using this method, and therefore it is a powerful informative tool in the process of OSAS diagnosis [21]. For a video example of the DISE, please visit Chap. 6 (Video 6.1).

From the physical exam, the clinician obtains a general sense of the airway collapse as well as the patient's particular features that occur during sleep.

3.6 Further Investigations: Sleep Study

To diagnose the disorder definitively, it is invaluable to observe the disease in action—that is to say, over a period where the patient is naturally sleeping. Most clinics will administer a sleep study, of which there are multiple types.

The sleep studies are generally divided into four levels, increasing in ease but decreasing in their comprehensiveness. Level 1, the polysomnography is the gold standard, but quite resource intensive and impractical as a screening tool. The higher levels are easy to administer at home but require interpretation by a specialist.

Level 1: The polysomnography (PSG) is done overnight in a sleep lab or hospital. It records your brain waves, heartbeats, and breathing as you sleep, whilst also charting eye and limb movements, and oxygen in your blood. This study is supervised by a technician or physician during the night. It is very comprehensive and can diagnose a multitude of sleep disorders.

Level 2: The same type of study is performed without a technician in attendance; it still allows a high degree of information but there no active observation.

Level 3: This type of study is conducted at home, and the device provided records oxygen levels, heart rate, airflow, snoring, and other parameters while asleep.

Level 4 refers to a screening test for sleep apnoea but with monitoring the oxygen level of the blood during sleep. During apnoea events, oxygen is not getting to the lungs and so isn't being exchanged into the blood. This would be reflected in the oximeter (or oxygen meter) reading, so the results might be useful for a physician in determining those who could have the condition. This study is usually used in children.

Level 3 and 4 are considered Home Sleep Studies (HSS), alternatives to the expensive PSG that monitors natural sleep throughout a night. A device is taken home and self-administered during sleep. It mainly measures breathing effort, air flow, and vitals, but is limited because it does not measure brain and heart activity like the PSG, which is important in accurately describing the sleep stage that the person is in. There are also subtle features of OSAS which the HSS is simply not sensitive enough to pick up, such as hypopnoeas [22]. Although it is cost effective and reliable for typical cases, a failed HSS should still be followed up by a PSG, according to the American Academy of Sleep Medicine [23].

Recently, several apps for the smartphone and devices have been developed to monitor sleep. They can roughly monitor sleep movement, snoring, and blood oxygen, which are useful parameters like those involved in the HSS. Most of these unfortunately lack scientific value, but they are developing rapidly, so this may change in the near future.

3.7   More About the Polysomnography

The PSG is a comprehensive exploration of a patient's sleep. You would expect to stay overnight at the clinic for one of these tests. It requires some preparation as the sleep needs to be as natural as possible: no prior sleeping or consumption of substances such as caffeine or alcohol. Every centre is slightly different but it is generally required to have not eaten anything from the afternoon of the night one takes the test. Devices such as electrodes, cameras, and sensors will be placed in the room and on the body to monitor sleep. The results will be interpreted in the morning.

See the appendix for a typical polysomnogram. Notice that information such as the position of sleeping and body movement is recorded—it is important to determine this seemingly superfluous information, as it may be the case that apnoea only occurs in a specific position or is complicated by other conditions such as Periodic Limb Movement disorders (PLM).

3.8 Conclusion

Sleep apnoea is challenging to notice, and when it is, the disease has likely already impacted the patient's quality of life significantly. If, however, we are aware of the risk factors and seek medical help at the earliest suspicions, we can prevent this harm. The ease and affordability of diagnosis is increasing rapidly with the development of technology and increased research efforts: it is not unreasonable to see the home diagnosis reaching the accuracy of the laboratory PSG in the coming years.

So, we have discussed the pathophysiology of OSAS, what the risk factors are, and how it is diagnosed. The following chapters will discuss the non-surgical and surgical treatments of the syndrome.

References

1. Bickelmann AG, Burwell CS, Robin ED, Whaley RD. Extreme obesity associated with alveolar hypoventilation; a Pickwickian syndrome. Am J Med. 1956;21:811–8. https://doi.org/10.1016/0002-9343(56)90094-8.
2. Pevernagie DA, et al. On the rise and fall of the apnea-hypopnea index: a historical review and critical appraisal. J Sleep Res. 2020;29:e13066. https://doi.org/10.1111/jsr.13066.
3. Lonergan RP 3rd, Ware JC, Atkinson RL, Winter WC, Suratt PM. Sleep apnea in obese miniature pigs. J Appl Physiol. 1998;1985(84):531–6. https://doi.org/10.1152/jappl.1998.84.2.531.

4. Hendricks JC, et al. The English bulldog: a natural model of sleep-disordered breathing. J Appl Physiol. 1987;1985(63):1344–50. https://doi.org/10.1152/jappl.1987.63.4.1344.

5. Punjabi NM. The epidemiology of adult obstructive sleep apnea. Proc Am Thorac Soc. 2008;5:136–43. https://doi.org/10.1513/pats.200709-155MG.

6. Senaratna CV, et al. Prevalence of obstructive sleep apnea in the general population: a systematic review. Sleep Med Rev. 2017;34:70–81. https://doi.org/10.1016/j.smrv.2016.07.002.

7. Cowan DC, Livingston E. Obstructive sleep apnoea syndrome and weight loss: review. Sleep Disord. 2012;2012:163296. https://doi.org/10.1155/2012/163296.

8. Krishnan V, Dixon-Williams S, Thornton JD. Where there is smoke... There is sleep apnea: exploring the relationship between smoking and sleep apnea. Chest. 2014;146:1673–80. https://doi.org/10.1378/chest.14-0772.

9. Simou E, Britton J, Leonardi-Bee J. Alcohol and the risk of sleep apnoea: a systematic review and meta-analysis. Sleep Med. 2018;42:38–46. https://doi.org/10.1016/j.sleep.2017.12.005.

10. McNicholas WT. Diagnosis of obstructive sleep apnea in adults. Proc Am Thorac Soc. 2008;5:154–60. https://doi.org/10.1513/pats.200708-118MG.

11. Taken K, Ekin S, Arisoy A, Gunes M, Donmez MI. Erectile dysfunction is a marker for obstructive sleep apnea. Aging Male. 2016;19:102–5. https://doi.org/10.3109/13685538.2015.1131259.

12. Loh NK, Dinner DS, Foldvary N, Skobieranda F, Yew WW. Do patients with obstructive sleep apnea wake up with headaches? Arch Intern Med. 1999;159:1765–8. https://doi.org/10.1001/archinte.159.15.1765.

13. Bestetti RB, Restini CB, Couto LB. Development of anatomophysiologic knowledge regarding the cardiovascular system: from Egyptians to Harvey. Arq Bras Cardiol. 2014;103:538–45. https://doi.org/10.5935/abc.20140148.

14. Osman EZ, Osborne J, Hill PD, Lee BW. The Epworth sleepiness scale: can it be used for sleep apnoea screening among snorers? Clin Otolaryngol Allied Sci. 1999;24:239–41. https://doi.org/10.1046/j.1365-2273.1999.00256.x.

15. Chung F, et al. STOP questionnaire: a tool to screen patients for obstructive sleep apnea. Anesthesiology. 2008;108:812–21. https://doi.org/10.1097/ALN.0b013e31816d83e4.

16. Chiu HY, et al. Diagnostic accuracy of the Berlin questionnaire, STOP-BANG, STOP, and Epworth sleepiness scale in detecting obstructive sleep apnea: a bivariate meta-analysis. Sleep Med Rev. 2017;36:57–70. https://doi.org/10.1016/j.smrv.2016.10.004.

17. Amra B, Rahmati B, Soltaninejad F, Feizi A. Screening questionnaires for obstructive sleep apnea: an updated systematic review. Oman Med J. 2018;33:184–92. https://doi.org/10.5001/omj.2018.36.
18. Johns MW. A new method for measuring daytime sleepiness: the Epworth sleepiness scale. Sleep. 1991;14(6):540–5. https://doi.org/10.1093/sleep/14.6.540.
19. Kline LR, Collop N, Finlay G. Clinical presentation and diagnosis of obstructive sleep apnea in adults. Philadelphia: Wolters Kluwer; 2021.
20. Nuckton TJ, Glidden DV, Browner WS, Claman DM. Physical examination: Mallampati score as an independent predictor of obstructive sleep apnea. Sleep. 2006;29:903–8. https://doi.org/10.1093/sleep/29.7.903.
21. Kotecha B, De Vito A. Drug induced sleep endoscopy: its role in evaluation of the upper airway obstruction and patient selection for surgical and non-surgical treatment. J Thorac Dis. 2018;10:S40–7. https://doi.org/10.21037/jtd.2017.10.32.
22. Rosen IM, et al. Clinical use of a home sleep apnea test: an updated American Academy of sleep medicine position statement. J Clin Sleep Med. 2018;14:2075–7. https://doi.org/10.5664/jcsm.7540.
23. Kapur VK, et al. Clinical practice guideline for diagnostic testing for adult obstructive sleep apnea: an American Academy of sleep medicine clinical practice guideline. J Clin Sleep Med. 2017;13:479–504. https://doi.org/10.5664/jcsm.6506.

The Non-Surgical Treatment of OSAS

4

Since the description of the disease in the 1960s, there have been many approaches to treat it. Each method will be explored, but they can generally be organised into non-surgical and surgical methods:

Non-surgical	Surgical
Behaviour modification	Bone surgery
Positive airway pressure	Soft tissue surgery
Oral appliances	Neurostimulation
Positional therapy	

These will be discussed in the current and the next chapter respectively.

4.1   Behaviour Modification

Multiple lifestyle changes have been proven to drastically reduce the severity of OSAS. The most significant of these is weight loss, which is recommended to all patients with obesity/weight-related OSAS. A reduction of weight by 10 kg has been found in some trials to reduce AHI by almost half [1].

© The Author(s), under exclusive license to Springer Nature Switzerland AG 2023
A. Shetty, P. M. Baptista Jardín, *A Patient's Guide to Obstructive Sleep Apnea Syndrome*, https://doi.org/10.1007/978-3-031-38264-2_4

Whether the loss of weight is achieved by a combination of diet and exercise, medication, or bariatric surgery (a surgical weight-loss operation), there will be a marked improvement in OSAS severity. This approach, however, is generally not a cure, and must be treated instead as a highly effective complement to a more primary intervention such as CPAP or OSAS-specific surgery.

4.2   Positive Airway Pressure

Positive airway pressure (PAP) is a technology that controls the rate of entry and escape of air into the body to maintain a pressure in the airway. As aforementioned, Colin Sullivan's utilisation of this technology in the treatment of OSAS in 1981 proved highly effective and is still the gold-standard treatment to this date [2].

There are two types of PAP: CPAP (continuous PAP) and BPAP (bilevel PAP, where a different pressure provided when breathing in and breathing out). Some patients may find it difficult to exhale against the CPAP or find it ineffective, in which case the latter might be more suitable as it can be further personalised.

CPAP is effective in suppressing apnoea events, boasting a near 90% decrease in AHI post-treatment [3], but it should be noted that the device must be worn every night and does not "cure" the disorder. Beyond an increased quality of sleep and a marked decrease in daytime sleepiness, CPAP treatment can improve cognitive function, decrease hypertension, and risk motor vehicle accidents. CPAP was not found to significantly reduce the cardiovascular event or stroke risk for sufferers of OSAS and only improved all-cause mortality[1] in middle-aged and elderly males.

---

[1] All-cause mortality refers to death by any cause. It is interesting that there is this disparity between the genders, and it is suggested to be due to the later onset lesser severity of OSAS seen in women as compared to men in general.

In general, the improvement of symptoms and quality of life is proportional to the severity of the individual case [4–10].

4.3   Administering PAP

Since the device must be used every night on the face, it must be comfortable. Although its correct use dramatically alleviates OSAS, multiple studies show that 30–80% of patients do not adhere to the treatment (≤ 4 h use per night), because of the uncomfortable side effects that may present [11].

Probably the most crucial aspect is the mask that will be in contact with the face. Each face is different, and there is a need for the mask to feel comfortable; there are three different face masks: nasal masks, oro-nasal masks, and nasal olives (see Fig. 4.1).[2]

The nasal mask only covers the nose. The oronasal mask is more extensive and covers the mouth and the nose.

The nasal olives are introduced and rest in the entrance of the nostrils.

Acclimatisation to the device is gradual as the mask can feel unnatural and different. The user's initial experience with the device is vital in promoting long-term continued use, and newer technologies and calibration methods have allowed clinicians to provide a more personalised and successful treatment strategy.

---

[2]You may see "full-face mask" used interchangeably with oro-nasal mask, and "nasal pillows" with nasal olives.

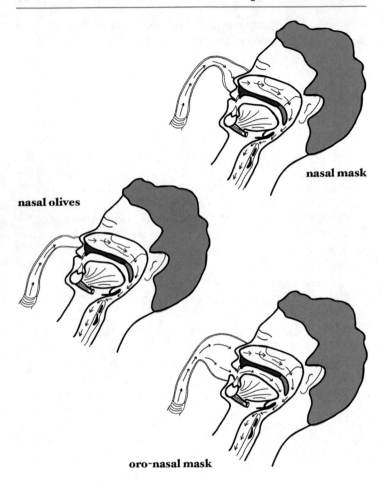

Fig. 4.1 Types of CPAP mask
Multiple factors will guide the choice of mask for patients, such as how they sleep (whether they move around a lot, sleep mainly on their back or side, etc.), how much pressure they require (the nasal mask is best for higher pressure settings and the oro-nasal mask leaks air the most), and whether other aspects hinder mask fitting such as facial hair, obstructions in the nose or mouth, or claustrophobia

4.4   Side Effects and Management

The side effects of CPAP may include:

- dryness of the nose and mouth,
- a "stuffy nose" and nosebleeds,
- irritation of the skin of the face,
- stuffy nose,
- a claustrophobic sensation,
- pressure sores,
- difficulty falling asleep.

However, the following practices are effective in combatting some of these issues [12, 13]:

- humidification of the air,
- careful selection and individual modelling of the mask,
- maintenance of the hygiene of the device,
- regular review with the patient's physician.

The final point is the most important—a close relationship between the patient and physician allows issues to be corrected early, improving long-term success.

Recently, the development of apps alongside the CPAP machines has supported the initiation of use and allows better access to information for the user and the healthcare provider regarding nightly use, tolerability, and management [14].

4.5   Oral Appliances

Oral appliances are growing in popularity as an alternative to PAP for those who find it ineffective or adhere poorly. These devices work by physically holding the airway open to suppress OSAS events during the night, by action either on the jaw or the tongue. These devices are slightly less effective than PAP and may cause permanent effects upon the anatomy of the upper airway. They also are only effective for two-thirds of patients due to the locality of their influence. However, the ease and comfort of the devices may provide a better overall treatment as they are better adhered to on average.

4.6   Mandibular Advancement Devices (MAD)

The mandible, or lower jaw, collapses back in most cases of OSAS. These devices help prevent this by holding the jaw in a forward position, thereby keeping the throat open for the passage of air (see Fig. 4.2). They usually attach to both sets of teeth and are adjustable to cater to different jaw types and sizes.

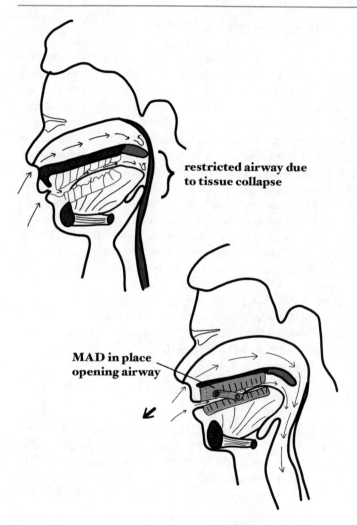

restricted airway due to tissue collapse

MAD in place opening airway

Fig. 4.2 Mandibular advancement devices
A mandibular advancement device is an effective solution for those with mild to moderate OSAS. These devices can be purchased over the counter or custom-made, but the concept is generally the same: using the upper jaw as an anchor, the lower jaw is held forward to prevent structures such as the base of the tongue collapsing into the throat. This encourages airflow

4.7   Tongue Retaining Devices

These work exactly as the name suggests, by slightly pulling the tongue forward so it does not collapse back into the throat. Though not as common as the MADs discussed above, they are still proven to be effective in the reduction of snoring and have a considerable effect on AHI as well [15].

Oral appliances are a good treatment for OSAS in certain patients, however CPAP is usually more effective. There are short- and long-term side effects with its use, which should be kept in mind. In the short term, the device will likely cause irritation, muscular pain, and problems with salivation; however, these are seen to disappear within the first few months. The long-term issue with a device holding the jaw in a certain position for an extended period is that the patient's jaw will adapt and change shape accordingly, so the device will need to be continually adjusted to be effective.

Studies show that the efficacy of such appliances decreases after 2–10 years, so it is not a permanent solution. The anatomy of the patient will also be changed after long-term use, such as the position of your teeth when biting [16].

4.8   Positional Therapy

OSAS events often occur when the patient is laying on their back as gravity aids in collapsing the throat. This can sometimes be fixed by lying on one's side. If the severity of the patient's OSAS depends on their position, they are said to have Positional Sleep Apnoea. Appropriate positioning can improve this condition by up to 60% [17].

An effective solution to Positional Sleep Apnoea is a small device that monitors position and uses minor stimuli to discourage the patient from sleeping on their back, reducing the number of events experienced during the night. They are easy to use, cost-effective, and do not present with significant side effects. Examples of these devices are included in Chap. 6.

Some smartphone apps have recently been created for this reason but require that the phone is worn on the body during sleep—in a pyjama pocket, for example. If you are facing upward and snoring, it will vibrate until you roll over to the side.

4.9 Conclusion

Though CPAP is the gold standard in OSAS treatment and is superior in the general case, certain patients such as those with mild to medium sleep apnoea, those who adhere poorly to CPAP, or those whose problem is specific and targetable, may find these alternative solutions convenient and cost-effective. Each OSAS patient nevertheless requires a thorough examination by a physician to decide on the treatment route, as it depends on many factors unique to each individual.

References

1. Smith PL, Gold AR, Meyers DA, Haponik EF, Bleecker ER. Weight loss in mildly to moderately obese patients with obstructive sleep apnea. Ann Intern Med. 1985;103:850–5. https://doi.org/10.7326/0003-4819-103-6-850.
2. Sullivan CE, Issa FG, Berthon-Jones M, Eves L. Reversal of obstructive sleep apnoea by continuous positive airway pressure applied through the nares. Lancet. 1981;1:862–5. https://doi.org/10.1016/s0140-6736(81)92140-1.
3. Patil SP, et al. Treatment of adult obstructive sleep apnea with positive airway pressure: an American Academy of sleep medicine systematic review, meta-analysis, and GRADE assessment. J Clin Sleep Med. 2019;15:301–34. https://doi.org/10.5664/jcsm.7638.
4. Jennum P, Tonnesen P, Ibsen R, Kjellberg J. Obstructive sleep apnea: effect of comorbidities and positive airway pressure on all-cause mortality. Sleep Med. 2017;36:62–6. https://doi.org/10.1016/j.sleep.2017.04.018.
5. Jennum P, Tonnesen P, Ibsen R, Kjellberg J. All-cause mortality from obstructive sleep apnea in male and female patients with and without continuous positive airway pressure treatment: a registry study with 10 years of follow-up. Nat Sci Sleep. 2015;7:43–50. https://doi.org/10.2147/NSS.S75166.

6. Antic NA, et al. The effect of CPAP in normalizing daytime sleepiness, quality of life, and neurocognitive function in patients with moderate to severe OSA. Sleep. 2011;34:111–9. https://doi.org/10.1093/sleep/34.1.111.

7. Patel SR, White DP, Malhotra A, Stanchina ML, Ayas NT. Continuous positive airway pressure therapy for treating sleepiness in a diverse population with obstructive sleep apnea: results of a meta-analysis. Arch Intern Med. 2003;163:565–71. https://doi.org/10.1001/archinte.163.5.565.

8. Guo J, et al. Effect of CPAP therapy on cardiovascular events and mortality in patients with obstructive sleep apnea: a meta-analysis. Sleep Breath. 2016;20:965–74. https://doi.org/10.1007/s11325-016-1319-y.

9. Horstmann S, Hess CW, Bassetti C, Gugger M, Mathis J. Sleepiness-related accidents in sleep apnea patients. Sleep. 2000;23:383–9.

10. Martinez-Garcia MA, et al. Effect of CPAP on blood pressure in patients with obstructive sleep apnea and resistant hypertension: the HIPARCO randomized clinical trial. JAMA. 2013;310:2407–15. https://doi.org/10.1001/jama.2013.281250.

11. Weaver TE, Grunstein RR. Adherence to continuous positive airway pressure therapy: the challenge to effective treatment. Proc Am Thorac Soc. 2008;5:173–8. https://doi.org/10.1513/pats.200708-119MG.

12. Pepin JL, et al. Side effects of nasal continuous positive airway pressure in sleep apnea syndrome. Study of 193 patients in two French sleep centers. Chest. 1995;107:375–81. https://doi.org/10.1378/chest.107.2.375.

13. Massie CA, Hart RW, Peralez K, Richards GN. Effects of humidification on nasal symptoms and compliance in sleep apnea patients using continuous positive airway pressure. Chest. 1999;116:403–8. https://doi.org/10.1378/chest.116.2.403.

14. Suarez-Giron M, et al. Mobile health application to support CPAP therapy in obstructive sleep apnoea: design, feasibility and perspectives. ERJ Open Res. 2020;6:00220. https://doi.org/10.1183/23120541.00220-2019.

15. Lazard DS, et al. The tongue-retaining device: efficacy and side effects in obstructive sleep apnea syndrome. J Clin Sleep Med. 2009;5:431–8.

16. Marklund M. Update on oral appliance therapy for OSA. Curr Sleep Med Rep. 2017;3:143–51. https://doi.org/10.1007/s40675-017-0080-5.

17. Srijithesh PR, Aghoram R, Goel A, Dhanya J. Positional therapy for obstructive sleep apnoea. Cochrane Database Syst Rev. 2019;5:CD010990. https://doi.org/10.1002/14651858.CD010990.pub2.

The Surgical Treatment of OSAS

5

On average, CPAP usage falls approximately 1 year after beginning, and some of the common reasons for this are: irritation from excessive pressure; the leakage of air; nasal obstruction or watery nose in the morning (rhinitis); or general discomfort and inconvenience in using the mask.

Surgical intervention can improve adherence to CPAP or treat the condition directly. It is considered an alternative treatment, however, as most improve without it. There are a variety of procedures, and the best course depends on the anatomy of the patient and the specifics of their condition.

As mentioned in the previous chapter, a visualisation of the upper airway is needed. A DISE (drug-induced sleep endoscopy), for example, allows the sleep physician to determine the specific areas of obstruction and thus the best course of surgery.

Supplementary Information The online version contains supplementary material available at https://doi.org/10.1007/978-3-031-38264-2_5. The videos can be accessed individually by clicking the DOI link in the accompanying figure caption or by scanning this link with the SN More Media App.

© The Author(s), under exclusive license to Springer Nature Switzerland AG 2023

A. Shetty, P. M. Baptista Jardín, *A Patient's Guide to Obstructive Sleep Apnea Syndrome*, https://doi.org/10.1007/978-3-031-38264-2_5

5.1   Nasal Surgery

Nasal problems are often related to abnormalities in the shape or anatomy of the nose, such as a deviated septum, large turbinates, nasal polyps, or chronic rhinosinusitis. See Fig. 3.5 to appreciate the potential problems in the nose again.

Addressing the nose with a surgical procedure can dramatically improve CPAP tolerance and, more importantly, its effectiveness. A recent study found that 90% of those who were not using CPAP before surgery subsequently adhered to or tolerated it after an isolated nasal surgical operation. They demonstrated a significant reduction in pressure from the machine and therefore greater comfort in its use. Furthermore, they found a 40% increase in the number of hours that the CPAP machine was used [1].

Nasal surgery alone does not cure OSAS but results in a reduction of the AHI in many cases, leading to an improvement in the quality of life reported by sleepiness questionnaires [2–6].

5.2   Tonsil and Adenoid Surgery

The enlargement of the tonsils and adenoids (Fig. 5.1) creates significant obstruction in the airway. These tissues are particularly prominent in children, so tonsillectomy and adenoidectomy (the surgical reduction or removal of the tonsils and adenoids) are usually the first choices in the treatment of children with OSAS.

Although these tissues reduce in size with age, such procedures may still be required for adults with persisting tonsil and adenoid enlargement, but usually in combination with other procedures in the upper airway [7].

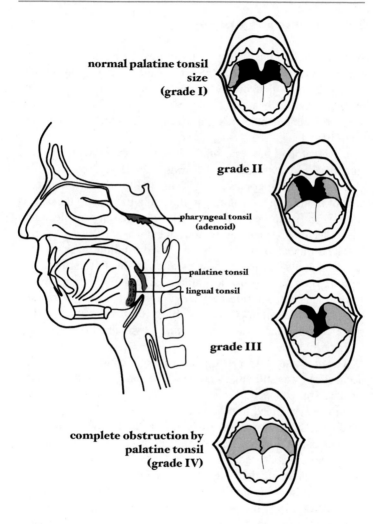

Fig. 5.1 Various tonsils and sizes

Notice the three tonsils in the throat. When entering from the nose, you encounter the pharyngeal tonsils also known as the adenoids. Further down, at the back of the mouth, there are the palatine tonsils which are the ones we commonly just call "tonsils". Under these is the lingual tonsil, which really is just the back part of the tongue. Any of these can become enlarged and block the airway causing OSAS. Notice the different grades of palatine tonsil size and the subsequent constriction of the back of the throat. As these enlarge, it becomes significantly more difficult to breathe from the mouth

5.3   Palate Surgery

As mentioned in the history, prior to the invention of CPAP, the only effective treatment for OSAS was the tracheostomy—a surgical procedure that involved creating a hole in the windpipe from the front of the neck. It is now considered a last resort treatment at this moment, as it significantly affects the patient's quality of life.

It was around the time of the invention of CPAP that a new surgical intervention was developed: the Uvulopalatopharyngoplasty (UPPP or UP3 for short), which consists of modifying the palate and the uvula to open up the airway (Fig. 5.3). It can be performed with or without tonsillectomy/adenoidectomy, depending on the patient.

The aim was to prevent the uvula from falling back into the airway and obstructing airflow by altering the soft tissue in that region. The results were not initially successful, helping only a few patients with snoring for a short period. The only permanent effect of initial attempts was a slight improvement in AHI in some cases. Other cases were actually worsened due to tissue scarring.

The procedure underwent multiple modifications over the next decades but was still amply criticized by many non-surgical physicians. This changed, however, in the early 2000s when the procedure was extended to modify the lateral walls avoiding cutting off the uvula, which improved the results, lessened the damage to the soft palate, and avoided complications. See Fig. 5.2 for the evolution of this procedure.

Although the modern UPPP is not a definite cure for OSAS, it does lower the AHI, significantly improving the patient's quality of life. Nowadays, the procedure and its modifications are often incorporated in one surgical treatment consisting of multi-level procedures (i.e., combined with a procedure on the nose, tongue base, tonsils, etc.) [8–18].

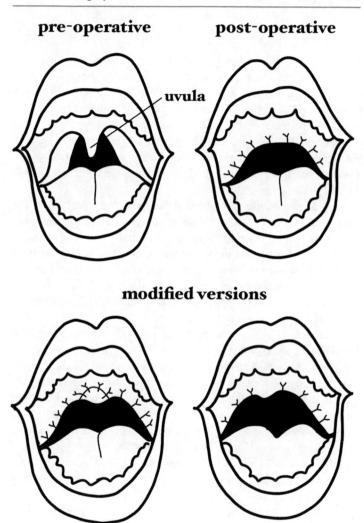

Fig. 5.2 Uvulopalatopharyngoplasty (UPPP)
The top-left diagram shows the normal airway with uvula and palate intact. The traditional operation removed the uvula completely and modified the soft palate, shown as the top-right diagram. More modern developments are shown subsequently: at bottom-left, the modified UPPP aims to tighten the tissues in the region without cutting much out. At bottom left, an approach conserving the uvula with minimal modification is pictured

5.4   Tongue Surgery

The tongue is quite a unique structure in the body in that it is formed by diverse muscles and has an extensive range of movement. To support this, it is suspended in the mouth and is not entirely fixed to any bony structure (partially to the mandible and hyoid bone—which itself is also "floating"—see Fig. 5.3).

As a result, a tongue that is enlarged or with lack of muscle tone tend to fall back into the throat during sleep, obstructing the airway. The enlargement of the base of the tongue can also cause this, as pictured opposite.

Several procedures have been developed to try and avoid the collapsing of the tongue, such as mandibular advancement surgery. This can be done in two ways, the first is a process called traction which includes using special screws and threads to pull forward the lower jaw and suspend the tongue. The second procedure is called genioglossus advancement (see Fig. 5.3), performed by making a small cut in the lower jaw and inserting a piece of bone that helps pull the tongue forward.

Another way to alleviate this condition is to reduce the volume of the tongue itself, which can be done in two ways: resection and coblation. Resection involves cutting away a part of the tongue and is usually performed on the base of the tongue and is a highly specialised surgery, often requiring robots such as the Da Vinci surgical robot, and specialised training. It can also be performed down the midline of the tongue, where tissue is directly removed. The other way to reduce volume is called coblation, which is less invasive as it does not involve incisions. It is a radiofrequency device that heats and disintegrates parts of the tongue tissue, thus reducing its volume—see Fig. 5.4.

Recently, a very successful multilevel strategy has been developed involving radiofrequency with coblation or Robotic surgery on the tongue combined with palate reconstruction (from the previous part) has proven to be highly effective [19].

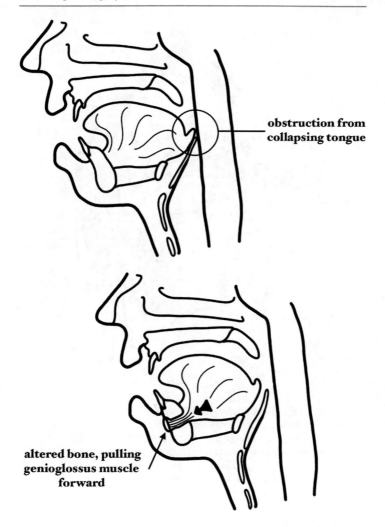

obstruction from collapsing tongue

altered bone, pulling genioglossus muscle forward

Fig. 5.3 Genioglossus advancement
The genioglossus muscle partially anchors the tongue to the front of the lower jaw. If the tongue regularly collapses into the back of the throat as is pictured in the top diagram, a modification of the jawbone can be made to thread the muscle through slightly, pulling the entire tongue forward with it and out of the throat

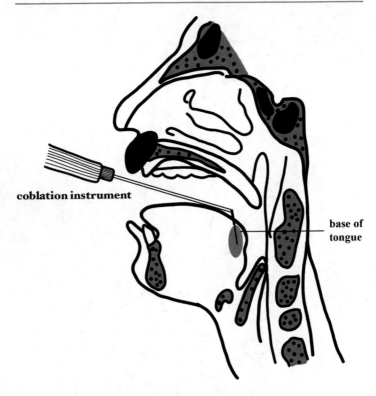

coblation instrument

base of
tongue

Fig. 5.4 Coblation of the base of the tongue
A specialised instrument uses radiofrequency plasma and a saline wash to dissolve tissue at the molecular level. It also produces fewer complications, heals quicker, and is less painful than traditional techniques. The soft palate can also be reduced with coblation if required, and this technique is often combined with multiple other procedures to provide a highly effective surgical solution to OSAS

5.5   Bony Frame Surgery

In more extreme cases or in patients where smaller procedures have failed to alleviate their condition, diverse procedures involving multiple regions of the facial skeleton may need to be performed to open up the airway.

What must be kept in mind is that their recovery time is often longer for such extensive procedures as the bones in the face are physically being reshaped. As well as this, the appearance of the patient may be altered.

An example of a combined procedure is the maxillomandibular advancement, or MMA, involving the movement of the upper and lower jaw (the maxilla and mandible respectively) forward, creating space behind the nose and tongue (Fig. 5.5). It can also be combined with genioglossus advancement, which has been mentioned previously.

MMA has been demonstrated to be one of the most effective surgical treatments for OSAS but is often only considered if other treatments have been ineffective (such as nasal surgeries, uvulopalatopharyngoplasty, tonsillectomy/adenoidectomy, tongue reduction, etc.), or in cases where deformities of the facial bones cause obstruction. Usually, an orthodontist is closely involved in repositioning the teeth and ensuring a comfortable bite after the surgery.

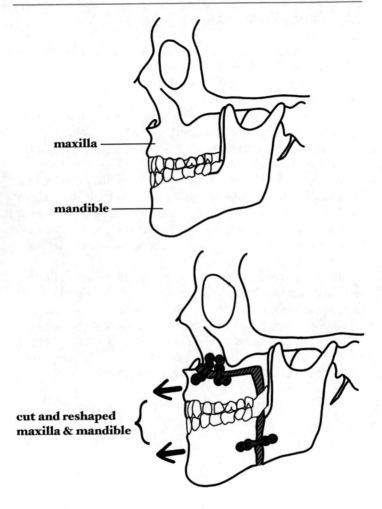

Fig. 5.5 Maxillomandibular advancement
*In this operation, the bony jaw, consisting of the mandible and maxilla as
pictured, is fully separated and reshaped. Titanium screws and plates are
used to fix the components into their new positions to heal. As can be seen,
this operation significantly increases the space in the mouth, which reduces
airway constriction*

5.6   Hypoglossal Nerve Stimulation

For some patients, CPAP is not effective, or they do not adhere to it. They may also not be fit for or desire anatomically modifying surgery. If, in addition, the cause of their OSAS is their tongue collapsing, with a loss of muscular tone, they may prefer Hypoglossal Nerve Stimulation (HNS). This is a recently developed treatment that has shown significant long-term improvements in patient's condition and quality of life with OSAS - all while leaving the facial tissue untouched.

The treatment works by implanting a device in the chest and/or in the chin that monitors breathing and electrically stimulates the nerve that controls the tongue (the hypoglossal nerve), encouraging it to move forward upon inhalation or in a cyclic way (Figs. 5.6, 5.7, 5.8, 5.9, and 5.10).

The device works while the patient is sleeping, and depending on the device the movement of the tongue is timed with the breathing of the patient. One can imagine how it can help unblock the airway when the patient breathes in, allowing the passage of air.

- There are specifications, however, for the type of patient for whom HNS is a valid treatment path. The patient should:
- Be older than 18 years.
- Have OSAS caused primarily by a collapsing tongue and palate (confirmed by a DISE, for example).
- Present with moderate to severe OSAS (an AHI range of 15–65 events per hour).
- Have shown intolerance or inadequate adherence to CPAP.
- Have a body mass index of less than 35.

These inclusion criteria are very simplified, and a complete evaluation of the patient including history, other medical conditions, specific anatomy, and other confounding factors must be carefully considered before this trajectory can be considered.

HNS has the advantage of being adjustable, which is essential for a chronic (long-term) condition like OSAS. Parameters such as the strength of the signal can be set exactly in a clinic or sleep

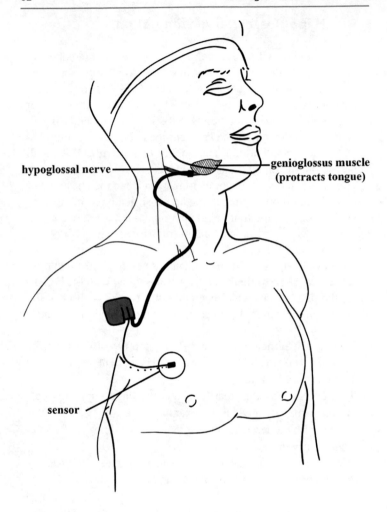

Fig. 5.6 Hypoglossal nerve stimulation
The sensor implanted in the chest detects breathing effort, and relays it to the computer pictured as the grey square on the patient's shoulder. This, in turn, stimulates the hypoglossal nerve implanted internally in order to stimulate the genioglossus muscle. When this muscle contracts, it pulls the tongue forward and therefore reopens the airway

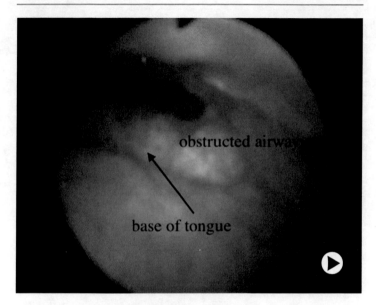

Fig. 5.7 HNS 1 (▶ https://doi.org/10.1007/000-b7v)

laboratory to optimize efficacy and comfort for the duration of treatment.

There are three different commercial implants available in the market at this moment: Inspire Medical Systems® (Inc., Maple Grove, MN), Imthera (LivaNova United Kingdom), and the (Nyxoah SA, Mont-Saint-Guibert, Belgium). All implants have shown outstanding results but act slightly differently, so each may prove to be more beneficial to different patients. Further information about the specific devices can be found in Chap. 6.

All patients being considered for HNS therapy must undergo a standard comprehensive sleep evaluation and an upper airway surgical consultation, which includes a normal endoscopy and a drug-induced sleep endoscopy (DISE).

There is an immense amount of information about HNS, and those further interested should seek advice from an ENT/sleep specialist [20–23].

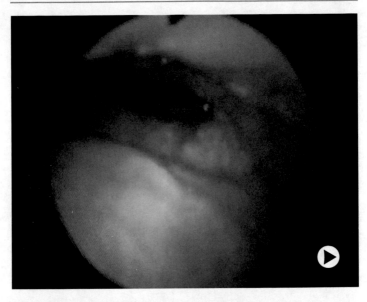

Fig. 5.8 HNS 2 (▶ https://doi.org/10.1007/000-b7t)

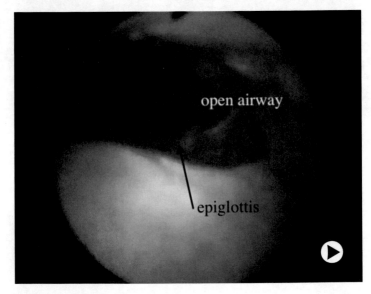

Fig. 5.9 HNS 3 (▶ https://doi.org/10.1007/000-b7s)

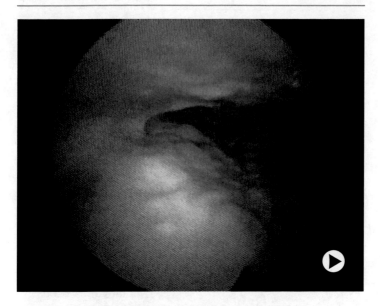

Fig. 5.10 HNS 4 (▶ https://doi.org/10.1007/000-b7w)

These are images from a video explanation of the Hypoglossal Nerve Stimulator implantation found in Chap. 6 (Video 6.2). Figure 5.7 shows the path of the device in the body, from the chest wall to the hypoglossal nerve near the tongue. Figure 5.8 shows the airway of a patient with an obstructed airway due to their tongue falling back into their throat. In Fig. 5.9, they are taking a breath, which is detected, and the tongue is stimulated. In Fig. 5.10, the stimulated tongue has moved forward and out of the way, allowing air to pass behind it

5.7 Tracheostomy

This procedure involves creating a hole in the windpipe (Fig. 5.11) that allows air to completely bypass the upper airway structures that block airflow. As aforementioned, the tracheostomy is the final alternative intervention to OSAS, reserved for those who do not tolerate any treatment.

Different studies have shown that a tracheostomy significantly improves AHI and daytime sleepiness in patients with OSAS, and other parameters such as blood pressure, arterial gases, the

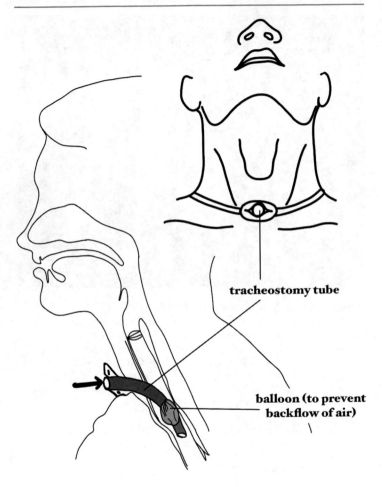

Fig. 5.11 Tracheostomy

A cut is made into the patient's windpipe and a tube is inserted as can be seen. The top diagram shows a securing device that can be worn around the neck to keep the tube in place. A balloon ensures that airflow is direct between the lungs and the outside without backflow, and therefore the air fully bypasses the mouth, nose, and throat

requirement for insulin, and mortality. Although the use of tracheostomy is less common in children, it has been found to be effective for those with severe OSAS stemming from complex conditions such as congenital disabilities or rare syndromes [24–29].

5.8   Conclusion

Although CPAP is considered the gold standard treatment, its efficacy and adherence in individual patients can be unpredictable. Surgical interventions can be considered in cases where it has failed, or the patient is unfit for it. However, it should be stressed again that since the condition presents very differently in every patient, finding the right treatment requires the consultation of experts and a process of trial and error.

The procedures that have been elaborated on in this chapter are OSAS are diverse and extensive. Since the field is relatively new, they are constantly enriched by innovation. We can expect to see further improvements in efficacy and patient outcomes in the near future.

References

1. Camacho M, et al. The effect of nasal surgery on continuous positive airway pressure device use and therapeutic treatment pressures: a systematic review and meta-analysis. Sleep. 2015;38:279–86. https://doi.org/10.5665/sleep.4414.
2. Wu J, et al. Apnea-hypopnea index decreased significantly after nasal surgery for obstructive sleep apnea: a meta-analysis. Medicine (Baltimore). 2017;96:e6008. https://doi.org/10.1097/MD.0000000000006008.
3. Hisamatsu K, Kudo I, Makiyama K. The effect of compound nasal surgery on obstructive sleep apnea syndrome. Am J Rhinol Allergy. 2015;29:e192–6. https://doi.org/10.2500/ajra.2015.29.4254.
4. Li HY, et al. Critical appraisal and meta-analysis of nasal surgery for obstructive sleep apnea. Am J Rhinol Allergy. 2011;25:45–9. https://doi.org/10.2500/ajra.2011.25.3558.
5. Li HY, et al. Improvement in quality of life after nasal surgery alone for patients with obstructive sleep apnea and nasal obstruction. Arch

Otolaryngol Head Neck Surg. 2008;134:429–33. https://doi.org/10.1001/archotol.134.4.429.

6. Stapleton AL, Chang YF, Soose RJ, Gillman GS. The impact of nasal surgery on sleep quality: a prospective outcomes study. Otolaryngol Head Neck Surg. 2014;151:868–73. https://doi.org/10.1177/0194599814544629.

7. Reckley LK, Fernandez-Salvador C, Camacho M. The effect of tonsillectomy on obstructive sleep apnea: an overview of systematic reviews. Nat Sci Sleep. 2018;10:105–10. https://doi.org/10.2147/NSS.S127816.

8. Browaldh N, Bring J, Friberg D. SKUP(3) RCT; continuous study: changes in sleepiness and quality of life after modified UPPP. Laryngoscope. 2016;126:1484–91. https://doi.org/10.1002/lary.25642.

9. Browaldh N, Nerfeldt P, Lysdahl M, Bring J, Friberg D. SKUP3 randomised controlled trial: polysomnographic results after uvulopalatopharyngoplasty in selected patients with obstructive sleep apnoea. Thorax. 2013;68:846–53. https://doi.org/10.1136/thoraxjnl-2012-202610.

10. Sommer UJ, et al. Tonsillectomy with Uvulopalatopharyngoplasty in obstructive sleep apnea. Dtsch Arztebl Int. 2016;113:1–8. https://doi.org/10.3238/arztebl.2016.0001.

11. Rotenberg BW, Theriault J, Gottesman S. Redefining the timing of surgery for obstructive sleep apnea in anatomically favorable patients. Laryngoscope. 2014;124(Suppl 4):S1–9. https://doi.org/10.1002/lary.24720.

12. Robinson S, et al. Upper airway reconstructive surgery long-term quality-of-life outcomes compared with CPAP for adult obstructive sleep apnea. Otolaryngol Head Neck Surg. 2009;141:257–63. https://doi.org/10.1016/j.otohns.2009.03.022.

13. Woodson BT, Steward DL, Weaver EM, Javaheri S. A randomized trial of temperature-controlled radiofrequency, continuous positive airway pressure, and placebo for obstructive sleep apnea syndrome. Otolaryngol Head Neck Surg. 2003;128:848–61. https://doi.org/10.1016/s0194-5998(03)00461-3.

14. Huang CC, et al. Improvement of baroreflex sensitivity in patients with obstructive sleep apnea following surgical treatment. Clin Neurophysiol. 2016;127:544–50. https://doi.org/10.1016/j.clinph.2015.05.022.

15. Peker Y, Hedner J, Norum J, Kraiczi H, Carlson J. Increased incidence of cardiovascular disease in middle-aged men with obstructive sleep apnea: a 7-year follow-up. Am J Respir Crit Care Med. 2002;166:159–65. https://doi.org/10.1164/rccm.2105124.

16. Weaver EM, Maynard C, Yueh B. Survival of veterans with sleep apnea: continuous positive airway pressure versus surgery. Otolaryngol Head Neck Surg. 2004;130:659–65. https://doi.org/10.1016/j.otohns.2003.12.012.

17. Haraldsson PO, Carenfelt C, Lysdahl M, Tingvall C. Does uvulopalato-pharyngoplasty inhibit automobile accidents? Laryngoscope. 1995;105:657–61. https://doi.org/10.1288/00005537-199506000-00019.

18. Tan KB, Toh ST, Guilleminault C, Holty JE. A cost-effectiveness analysis of surgery for middle-aged men with severe obstructive sleep apnea intolerant of CPAP. J Clin Sleep Med. 2015;11:525–35. https://doi.org/10.5664/jcsm.4696.

19. MacKay SG, Jefferson N, Grundy L, Lewis R. Coblation-assisted Lewis and MacKay operation (CobLAMO): new technique for tongue reduction in sleep apnoea surgery. J Laryngol Otol. 2013;127:1222–5. https://doi.org/10.1017/S0022215113002971.

20. Schwartz AR, et al. Therapeutic electrical stimulation of the hypoglossal nerve in obstructive sleep apnea. Arch Otolaryngol Head Neck Surg. 2001;127:1216–23. https://doi.org/10.1001/archotol.127.10.1216.

21. Strollo PJ Jr, et al. Upper-airway stimulation for obstructive sleep apnea. N Engl J Med. 2014;370:139–49. https://doi.org/10.1056/NEJMoa1308659.

22. Woodson BT, et al. Three-year outcomes of cranial nerve stimulation for obstructive sleep apnea: the STAR trial. Otolaryngol Head Neck Surg. 2016;154:181–8. https://doi.org/10.1177/0194599815616618.

23. Woodson BT, et al. Upper airway stimulation for obstructive sleep apnea: 5-year outcomes. Otolaryngol Head Neck Surg. 2018;159:194–202. https://doi.org/10.1177/0194599818762383.

24. Riley RW, Powell NB, Guilleminault C. Obstructive sleep apnea syndrome: a surgical protocol for dynamic upper airway reconstruction. J Oral Maxillofac Surg. 1993;51:742–7; discussion 748-749. https://doi.org/10.1016/s0278-2391(10)80412-4.

25. Haapaniemi JJ, Laurikainen EA, Halme P, Antila J. Long-term results of tracheostomy for severe obstructive sleep apnea syndrome. ORL J Otorhinolaryngol Relat Spec. 2001;63:131–6. https://doi.org/10.1159/000055728.

26. Coccagna G, Mantovani M, Brignani F, Parchi C, Lugaresi E. Tracheostomy in hypersomnia with periodic breathing. Bull Physiopathol Respir (Nancy). 1972;8:1217–27.

27. Bhimaraj A, Havaligi N, Ramachandran S. Rapid reduction of antihypertensive medications and insulin requirements after tracheostomy in a patient with severe obstructive sleep apnea syndrome. J Clin Sleep Med. 2007;3:297–9.

28. Camacho M, et al. Tracheostomy as treatment for adult obstructive sleep apnea: a systematic review and meta-analysis. Laryngoscope. 2014;124:803–11. https://doi.org/10.1002/lary.24433.

29. Rizzi CJ, et al. Tracheostomy for severe pediatric obstructive sleep apnea: indications and outcomes. Otolaryngol Head Neck Surg. 2017;157:309–13. https://doi.org/10.1177/0194599817702369.

Appendix: Links to Further Information

For examples of devices that aid with the alleviation of Positional Sleep Apnoea, see the following:

- Night balance (Philips, Netherlands).
- Night Shift (Advanced Brain Monitoring Inc. Carlsbad, California, USA).
- Somnibel (Sibelmed, Barcelona, Spain).
- iRollover (Snoremart, Belleview, Washington, USA).

The first three use vibration to elicit movement, and the last one is an acoustic signal.

Included is a video of the Drug-Induced Sleep Endoscopy demonstrating the collapse of the airway (Video 6.1).

Included is also a video of the Hypoglossal Nerve Stimulation device working in a patient with OSAS. Notice that when activated, the tongue is pushed forward, opening the airway. The video also shows the action of CPAP in opening the airway (Video 6.2).

Supplementary Information The online version contains supplementary material available at https://doi.org/10.1007/978-3-031-38264-2_6. The videos can be accessed individually by clicking the DOI link in the accompanying figure caption or by scanning this link with the SN More Media App.

© The Author(s), under exclusive license to Springer Nature Switzerland AG 2023

A. Shetty, P. M. Baptista Jardín, *A Patient's Guide to Obstructive Sleep Apnea Syndrome*, https://doi.org/10.1007/978-3-031-38264-2_6

For further information regarding Hypoglossal Nerve Stimulation products:

Imthera (https://www.livanova.com/).
Inspire (https://www.inspiresleep.com/).
Nyxoah (https://www.nyxoah.com/).

6.1 Polysomnogram (Fig. 6.1)

There are many channels of information:

CHIN, CHEST, ABD, LAT, and RAT are all measures of movement of the body. The chin, chest, abdomen, and left and right limbs, respectively. This helps interpret breathing effort, and restlessness. POS then furthermore lets us know if the patient is on their side, back, or face-down.

X—A1/2 (the first 8 leads except for CHIN) represent brain electrical activity.

FLOW represents the nasal air flow, and you can see that when it stops (an apnoea event) the chest, abdomen, and limb activity increase rapidly as the patient is trying desperately to breathe. Brain activity is also seen to increase as the body must wake up to reengage the airway muscles in order to breathe again.

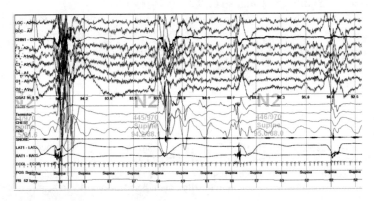

Fig. 6.1 PSG
Polysomnogram, or complete night study type 1

Printed in the United States
by Baker & Taylor Publisher Services